Quick & Tasty Keto Diet Recipes

A Low Carb Cookbook to Kickstart Your Body Transformation and Burn Fat Immediately | Carnivorous Recipes

Jane Leaner

Please note the information contained within this document is for educational and entertainment purposes only. All effort has been executed to present accurate, up to date, and reliable, complete information. No warranties of any kind are declared or implied. Readers acknowledge that the author is not engaging in the rendering of legal, financial, medical, or professional advice. The content within this book has been derived from various sources. Please consult a licensed professional before attempting any techniques outlined in this book.

By reading this document, the reader agrees that under no circumstances is the author responsible for any losses, direct or indirect, which are incurred as a result of the use of the information contained within this document, including, but not limited to, - errors, omissions, or inaccuracies.

Table of Content

—

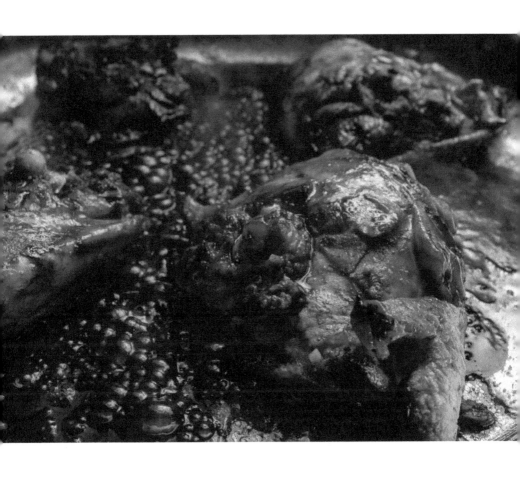

1.   Balsamic Chicken Thighs

Preparation time: 5 minutes

Cooking time: 20 minutes

Servings: 4

Ingredients:

- 4 (6 ounces) boneless chicken thighs (skinless)

- 2 teaspoons of seasoning (or use a mixture of garlic, salt, onion, pepper, and parsley)

- 4 tablespoons of "Balsamic mosto cotto" (or use balsamic reduction)

- ¼ cup of chicken broth (low sodium)

- 4 cups of steamed broccoli florets (crisp-tender)

Directions:

1. Season the chicken legs.

2. Grease the pan with non-stick cooking spray and set over high heat.

3. When it starts to glow, add the chicken, and reduce the heat to medium heat.

4. Cook each side for about 7 minutes or until cooked through.

5. Remove the chicken and set aside.

6. Add the broth and balsamic vinegar to the pan and scrape all the brown bits into the bottom of the pan.

7. Once the sauce has reduced by half, return the broccoli and chicken to the pan and toss to coat completely.

8. Serve immediately and enjoy. Good lunch!

Nutrition: Calories 314, Fat 10,8, Fiber 2,4, Carbs 8,8, Protein 43,6.

2.   Balsamic Chicken Veggies

Preparation Time: 5 minutes

Cooking Time: 25 minutes

Servings: 4

Ingredients:

- 1 ½ pound Boneless chicken thighs (skinless) -
- 1 tablespoon of Tuscan seasoning (or use a mixture of garlic, salt, parsley, pepper, garlic powder, red pepper, and onion)
- 4 tablespoon of Balsamic
- 1 tablespoon of Dijon mustard
- 2 cups of cherry/grape tomatoes (halved)
- 2 cups of zucchini (sliced into 3/8-inch slices)
- 1/3 cup of water

Directions:

1. In a large bowl, add the mustard, balsamic vinegar, and dressing and whisk together.

2. Then add the chicken and mix well.

3. Refrigerate to marinate, about 20 minutes to 8 hours.

4. Preheat the oven to 425 degrees.

5. Heat a cast-iron skillet over medium-high heat, shake off the excess marinade and place the chicken in the pan.

6. Cook for about 5 minutes on each side or until seared.

7. Meanwhile, sprinkle the vegetables around the pan and season with a pinch of salt and pepper.

8. Add the water to the marinade remaining in the bowl and mix well, then pour it over the vegetables and mix everything.

9. Transfer to the oven and cook for another 15 min.

10. Remove from the oven and serve!

Nutrition: Calories 280, Fat 9,9, Fiber 1,9, Carbs 7,5, Protein 38,7.

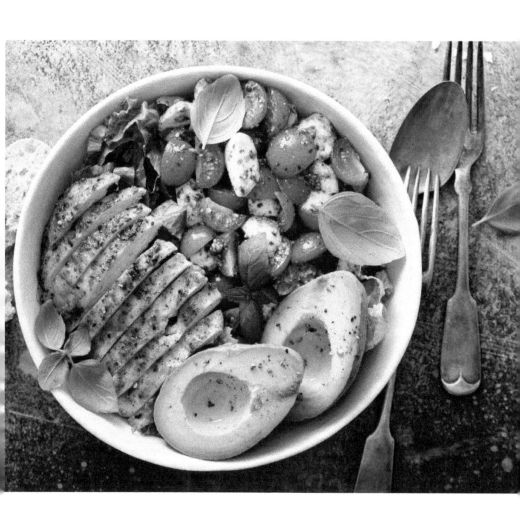

3. Basil Caprese Chicken

Preparation Time: 10 minutes

Cooking Time: 30 minutes

Servings: 4

Ingredients:
- 4 (6 oz each) of boneless chicken breasts (skinless)
- 9-12 fresh basil leaves
- 2 cups of fresh tomato slices
- 4 tablespoons of freshly grated parmesan cheese
- 1 tablespoon of Tuscan seasoning

Directions:
1. Preheat the oven to 350 degrees.
2. On a support surface, arrange the slices of chicken breast and in the center of each slice put the basil, tomatoes, and Parmesan.
3. Roll up the chicken.
4. Place the chicken in the oven and sprinkle it with the Tuscan dressing.
5. Add the tomato slices, basil, and cheese to the rolled chicken.
6. Sprinkle more seasoning and bake for about 30 minutes, or until chicken is cooked through, then remove from the oven and serve.

Nutrition: Calories 249, Fat 7,1, Fiber 1,1, Carbs 3,8, Protein 40,2.

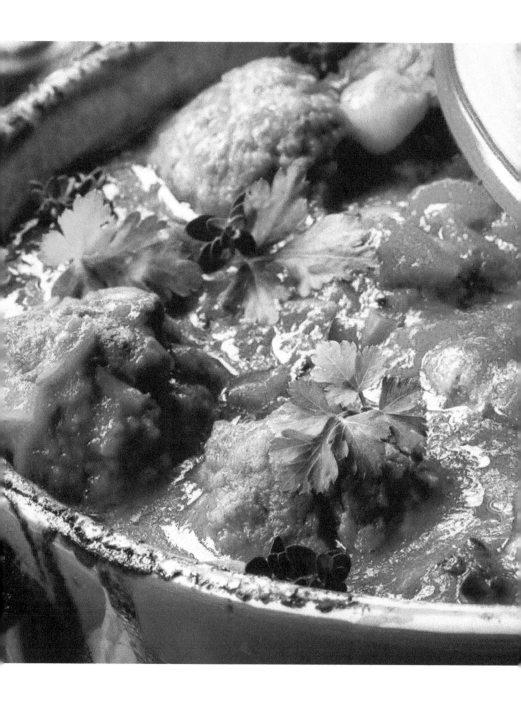

4.   Beef-Chicken Meatball Casserole

Preparation Time: 15 minutes

Cooking Time: 21 minutes

Servings: 7
Ingredients:

- 1 eggplant

- 10 oz. ground chicken

- 8 oz. ground beef

- 1 teaspoon of minced garlic

- 1 teaspoon of ground white pepper

- 1 tomato

- 1 egg

- 1 tablespoon of coconut flour

- 8 oz. Parmesan, shredded

- 2 tablespoon butter

- 1/3 cup cream

Directions:
1. Preheat the 360°F air fryer.

2. In a large bowl combine the minced chicken, minced meat, minced garlic, and minced white pepper, egg and mix thoroughly until well blended.

3. Add the coconut flour and mix.

4. With the mixture obtained, make small meatballs.

5. Sprinkle the fryer basket tray with butter and pour in the cream.

6. Peel the aubergines and chop them.

7. Put the meatballs on the cream and sprinkle with chopped aubergines.

8. Slice the tomato and place it on top of the aubergines, then make a layer of grated cheese on top of the sliced tomato.

9. Place the saucepan in the air fryer and cook for 21 minutes.

10. Let the saucepan cool to room temperature and then serve and enjoy!

Nutrition: Calories 314, Fat 16,8, Carbs 7,5, Protein 33,9.

5. Buffalo Chicken Sliders

Preparation Time: 10 minutes

Cooking Time: 15 minutes

Servings: 12

Ingredients:

- 2 lb Chicken breasts (cooked, shredded)
- 1 cup of wing sauce
- 1 pack of ranch dressing mix
- ¼ cup of blue cheese dressing (low fat)
- Lettuce (for topping)
- 12 buns (slider)

Directions:

1. Add the chicken breasts (shredded, cooked) in a large bowl along with the ranch dressing and wing sauce and stir well to incorporate.

2. Place a piece of lettuce onto each slider roll and top off using the chicken mixture.

3. Drizzle blue cheese dressing over chicken then top off using top buns of slider rolls and serve.

Nutrition: Calories 300, Fat 14.

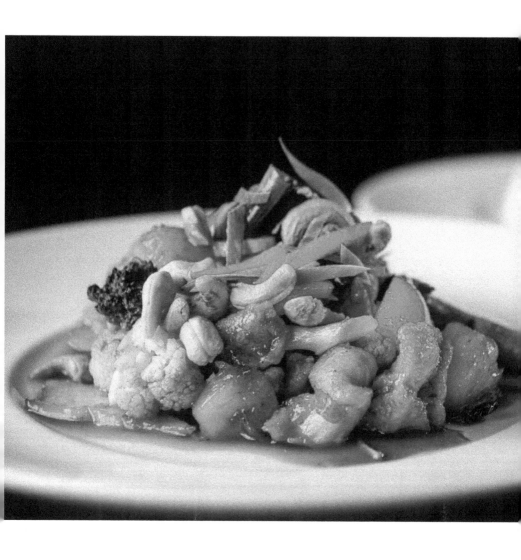

6.   Cashew Chicken

Preparation Time: 10 minutes

Cooking Time: 20 minutes

Servings: 4

Ingredients:

- 4 tsp of lemon or roasted garlic oil (or any other oil of choice)
- 1 ½ lbs of boneless chicken breast (skinless and sliced into thin strips)
- 1 tablespoon of Thai seasoning (or any mixture of onion, garlic, salt, red bell pepper, lemongrass, black pepper, chiles, and lime zest)
- 2 cups of green bell pepper (sliced into thin strips)
- 2 cups of red bell pepper (sliced into thin strips)
- 3 scallions (sliced - put the greens and whites separate)
- 24 cashews (chopped)

Directions:

1. In a skillet, heat the oil over medium-high heat.

2. Add the chicken strips to the pan and cook each side for about 5 minutes or until opaque.

3. Add the white shallot, peppers, and seasoning and mix thoroughly.

4. Close the lid and cook for another 7 minutes over high heat or until the chicken is cooked through, stirring occasionally.

---

5. Remove from the heat and sprinkle with the shallot and walnuts.

6. Serve hot and accompanied by cooked cauliflower if desired.

Nutrition: Calories 323, Fat 13,1, Fiber 2, Carbs 12,3, Protein 38,7.

7. Chicken and Kale Curry

Preparation Time: 20 minutes

Cooking Time: 1 hour

Servings: 3

Ingredients:

- 250 ml boiling water,
- 7 oz. of skinless and boneless chicken thighs
- 2 tablespoons of ground turmeric
- 1 tablespoon of olive oil,
- 1 red onion (diced)
- 1 Bird's eye chili (finely chopped)
- ½ tablespoon freshly chopped ginger
- ½ tablespoon of curry powder
- 1 ½ cloves garlic (crushed)
- 1 cardamom pods
- 100 ml of tinned coconut milk, light
- 2 cups of chicken stock
- 1 cup of tinned chopped tomatoes

Directions:

1. Put the chicken legs in a non-metallic bowl, add a tablespoon of turmeric and a teaspoon of olive oil, mix and set aside to marinate for approx. 30 minutes.

2. Fry the chicken legs over medium heat for about 5 minutes until cooked through and golden on all sides, then remove from the pan and set aside.

3. Add the remaining oil to a skillet over medium heat and add the onion, ginger, garlic, and chili.

4. Fry for about 10 minutes until soft.

5. Add a tablespoon of turmeric and half a tablespoon of curry powder to the pan and cook for another 2 minutes.

6. Add the cardamom pods, coconut milk, tomatoes, and chicken broth, and simmer for thirty minutes.

7. Once the sauce has reduced a little in the pan, add the chicken and kale and cook until the cabbage is tender and the chicken is hot enough.

8. Serve with buckwheat and garnish with chopped cilantro.

Nutrition: Calories 313, Fat 6, Carbs 23, Protein 13.

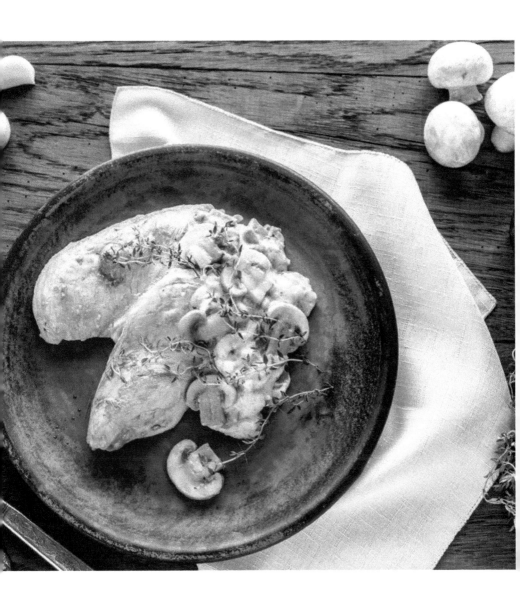

8.   Chicken and Mushrooms

Preparation Time: 10 minutes

Cooking Time: 15 minutes

Servings: 6
Ingredients:

- 2 chicken breasts

- 1 cup of sliced white champignons

- 1 cup of sliced green chilies

- ½ cup of scallions hacked

- 1 teaspoon of chopped garlic

- 1 cup of low-fat cheddar shredded cheese (1-1,5 lb. grams fat / ounce)

- 1 tablespoon of olive oil

- 1 tablespoon of butter

Directions:

1. Fry the chicken breasts with olive oil.

2. Season the chicken breasts with salt and pepper and then grill them on a grill plate.

3. In a pan, melt the butter and mix in the mushrooms, green peppers, shallots, and garlic until smooth.

4. Place the chicken on an oven dish, pour the mushroom mixture over it and cover with ham and cheese.

5. Place in the oven at 350 degrees until the cheese melts.

6. Remove from the oven and enjoy! Good lunch!

Nutrition: Calories 249 - Fat 11, Carbs 2, Protein 23.

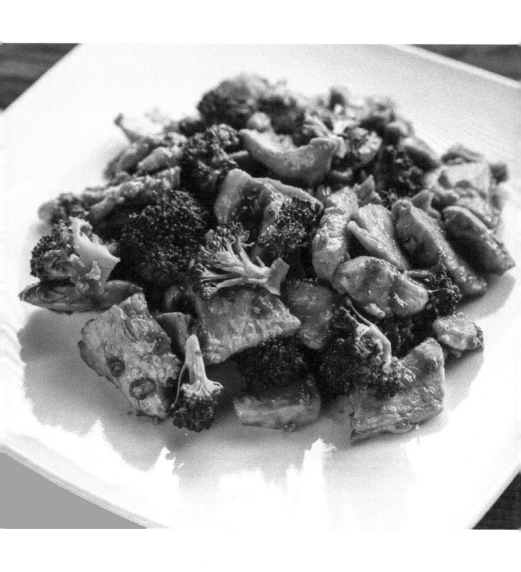

9.   Chicken Broccoli

Preparation Time: 5 minutes

Cooking Time: 30 minutes

Servings: 4

Ingredients:

- 4 cups of broccoli (cut into 1-inch pieces)
- 1 tablespoon of garlic gusto (or garlic and spring onion) seasoning)
- 1 ¼ pound (20 oz) of chicken thighs
- 1 tablespoon of chicken seasoning (or use a mixture of garlic, paprika, pepper, onion, salt)

Directions:

1. Preheat the oven to 350 degrees.

2. In a baking dish, add the chopped broccoli and chicken legs and sprinkle with the garlic dressing.

3. Cook for about 30 minutes or until the chicken is fully cooked.

4. Remove from the oven and serve.

Nutrition: Calories 271, Fat 13,3, Fiber 2,4, Carbs 6, Protein 22,6.

10.   Chicken Caper Sauce

Preparation Time: 5 minutes

Cooking Time: 25 minutes

Servings: 4

Ingredients:

- 2 pounds of boneless chicken tenderloins (skinless, and excess fat removed)
- 1 tablespoon of garlic and spring onion seasoning (or use a mixture of garlic, lemon, chives, sea salt, and parsley)
- ½ cup of chicken broth (low sodium)
- 2 tablespoons of fresh lemon juice
- 4 tablespoons of capers
- 2 tablespoons of butter (not margarine)
- Ground pepper and natural sea salt to taste

Directions:

1. At the bottom of an Instant Pot, place the chicken in a single layer.

2. Add the broth, lemon juice, and garlic dressing to a bowl and whisk together.

3. Pour the mixture over the chicken and sprinkle with the capers.

4. Close the lid, seal the valve, and cook over high heat for 10 min.

5. When done, quickly release the pressure, remove the chicken from the pot, and set it aside.

6. Set to Saute and bring the liquid to a boil.

7. Add the butter and whisk together and let the sauce cook until the liquid has reduced by half.

8. Turn off the pot and spread the sauce over the chicken; season with salt and pepper, serve, and enjoy!

Nutrition: Calories 265, Fat 5,9, Fiber 0,3, Carbs 0,6, Protein 48,3.

11. Chicken Coconut Poppers

Preparation Time: 10 minutes

Cooking Time: 10 minutes

Servings: 6

Ingredients:

- ½ cup of coconut flour

- 1 teaspoon of chili flakes

- 1 teaspoon of ground black pepper

- 1 teaspoon of garlic powder

- 11 oz. chicken breast, boneless, skinless

- 1 tablespoon of olive oil

Directions:

1. Preheat the air fryer to 365 F.

2. Cut the chicken breast into large enough cubes and place them in a large bowl.

3. Sprinkle the chicken cubes with chili flakes, ground black pepper, garlic powder and mix well with your hands.

4. Next, sprinkle the chicken cubes with the coconut flour and gently shake the bowl with the chicken cubes to coat the meat.

5. Grease the air fryer basket tray with olive oil and place the chicken cubes inside.

6. Cook the chicken poppers for 10 minutes.

7. Turn the chicken poppers after 5 minutes of cooking.

8. Allow cooked chicken poppers to cool, serve, and enjoy!

Nutrition: Calories 123, Fat 4,6, Carbs 6,9, Protein 13,2.

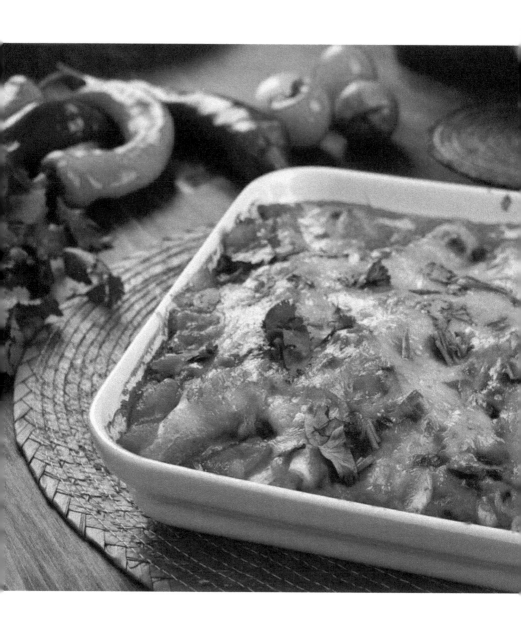

12.   Chicken Enchilada Bake

Preparation Time: 20 minutes

Cooking Time: 50 minutes

Servings: 5
Ingredients:

- 5 oz. Shredded chicken breast (boil and shred ahead) or 99 percent fat-free white chicken can be used in a pan.

- 1 can tomato paste

- 1 low sodium chicken broth can be fat-free

- 1/4 cup cheese with low-fat mozzarella

- 1 tablespoon of oil

- 1 tbsp. of salt

- Ground cumin, chili powder, garlic powder, oregano, and onion powder (all to taste)

- 1 to 2 zucchinis sliced longways (similar to lasagna noodles) into thin lines

- Sliced (optional) olives

Directions:

1. In a saucepan, heat the olive oil over medium/high heat.

2. Incorporate the tomato paste and seasonings and heat in the chicken broth for 2-3 minutes.

3. Stir regularly until boiling, then lower the heat for 15 min and then, set aside and cool to room temperature.

4. Meanwhile, put the courgettes in the enchilada sauce and place them on the bottom of a small pan.

5. Add just under ¼ cup of enchilada sauce to the chicken and mix.

6. In the pan with the zucchini, add the chicken and sprinkle it with bacon.

7. Add another layer of shredded zucchini with the enchilada sauce.

8. Continue to alternate the layers (similar to making lasagna) and finally cover with the remaining cheese and olives on top.

9. Bake for 35-40 minutes and when the cheese begins to brown, cover with aluminum foil.

Nutrition: Calories 312, Fat 10,2, Carbs 21,3, Protein 27.

13. Chicken Goulash

Preparation Time: 10 minutes

Cooking Time: 20 minutes

Servings: 6

Ingredients:

- 4 oz. chive stems

- 2 green peppers, chopped

- 1 teaspoon of olive oil

- 14 oz. ground chicken

- 2 tomatoes

- ½ cup of chicken stock

- 2 garlic cloves, sliced

- 1 teaspoon of salt

- 1 teaspoon of ground black pepper

- 1 teaspoon of mustard

Directions:

1. Preheat the air fryer to 365°F.

2. Spray the olive oil on the air fryer basket tray.

3. Coarsely chop the chives and place them in the pan in the air fryer basket.

4. Add the chopped green pepper and cook the vegetables for 5 minutes, then add the ground chicken.

5. Chop the tomatoes into small cubes, add them to the air fryer mixture and cook the mixture for another 6 minutes.

6. Add the chicken stock, sliced garlic cloves, salt, ground black pepper, mustard, and mix well.

7. Cook the goulash for another 6 minutes, then serve and enjoy.

Nutrition: Calories 161, Fat 6,1, Carbs 6, Protein 20,3.

14.   Chicken Mushroom Primavera

Preparation Time: 15 minutes

Cooking Time: 20 minutes

Servings: 4

Ingredients:

- 1 ½ pounds of boneless chicken breast (skinless, and excess fat removed)
- 1 tablespoon of chicken seasoning (or use any other seasoning you like)
- 1 cup of garden or cherry tomatoes (freshly chopped)
- 1 cup of fresh broccoli (chopped)
- 1 cup of fresh mushrooms (chopped)
- 1 cup of fresh green beans (chopped)
- 2 cups of cooked zucchini noodles
- 1 tablespoon of garlic and spring onion seasoning (or use a mixture of onion, fresh garlic, parsley, lemon)
- 2/3 cup of chicken broth (low sodium)
- 2 tablespoons of butter (not margarine)
- Ground pepper and natural sea salt - to taste

Directions:

1. Grease your pan with nonstick cooking spray and heat over medium-high heat.

2. Sprinkle both sides of the chicken with the chicken seasoning and add it to the pan.

3. Cook each side for about 10 min, or until it's well cooked.

FOR THE PRIMAVERA:

4. Grease another pan with the nonstick cooking spray and heat over medium heat.

5. Add all the vegetables with the garlic seasoning (except noodles), and saute for 5 minutes.

6. Add the chicken broth and increase the heat to high and bring the mixture to a boil.

7. Continue cooking until the liquid is reduced by half, then remove the pan from the heat.

8. Add the butter and stir well.

9. Heat the noodles in another pan.

10. Scoop the sauce and veggies onto the noodles, top with chicken, serve, and enjoy!

Nutrition: Calories 257, Fat 7,5, Fiber 2,9, Carbs 7,7.

15. Chicken Primavera

Preparation Time: 15 minutes

Cooking Time: 30 minutes

Servings: 4

Ingredients:
- 1 3/4 lb of boneless chicken breast (skinless)
- 7 cups of fresh vegetables (chopped)
- 4 tsp of toasted garlic oil (or any oil of choice)
- 1 tablespoon of garlic gusto seasoning (or any other seasoning you prefer)
- 1 tablespoon of salt and pepper seasoning

Directions:
1. Preheat the oven to 400 degrees.

2. Peel and chop the vegetables into 1-inch pieces.

3. Transfer the vegetables to a bowl along with the chicken, oil, and seasonings and mix until smooth.

4. Put the mixture in the pan and bake for about 30 min.

5. Halfway through cooking, turn them.

6. Remove from the oven, allow to cool for a while, serve hot and enjoy!

Nutrition: Calories 262, Fat 9, Fiber 2,9, Carbs 6,4, Protein 37,5.

16.   Chicken Salad with Pineapple and Pecans

Preparation Time: 10 minutes

Cooking Time: 5 minutes

Servings: 4

Ingredients:

- 6-ounce boneless, skinless, cooked, and cubed chicken breast

- Celery

- ¼ cup of pineapple

- ¼ cup orange, peeled segments

- 1 Tablespoon of pecans

- ¼ cup seedless grapes

- Salt and black chili pepper, to taste

- Cups cut from roman lettuce

Directions:

1. Into a bowl, place the chicken, celery, pineapple, grapes, pecans, and raisins.

2. Stir with a spoon until the mixture is combined, then season with salt and pepper.

3. On a plate, arrange a bed of lettuce, cover with the chicken mixture, and serve.

Nutrition: Calories 368, Fat 19, Carbs 20, Protein 25.

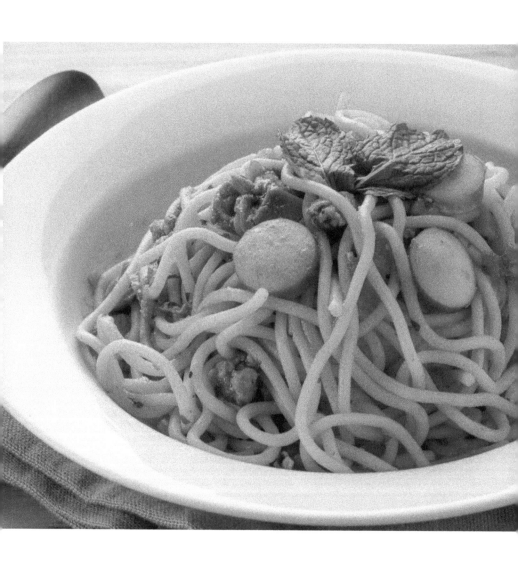

17. Chicken Sausage Spaghetti

Preparation Time: 10 minutes

Cooking Time: 15 minutes

Servings: 4

Ingredients:
- 4 cups of zucchini (spiraled)
- 1 ½ pound (24 oz) lean chicken sausage (or use beef sausage or turkey sausage)
- 1 tablespoon of Tuscan seasoning (or bell a mixture of garlic, bell pepper, parsley, black pepper, onion, and salt)
- 2 cups of Tomato sauce (no added sugar)
- 8 tablespoons of fresh Parmesan cheese (grated)

Directions:
1. Cut the chicken sausage into ½ inch pieces.

2. Place the pieces in a skillet and cook over medium-high heat for about 8 minutes or until golden, stirring occasionally.

3. Add the Tuscan dressing and tomato sauce to the pan and mix well to coat completely.

4. Increase the heat to high and bring the mixture to a boil, for about 4 min.

5. Add the noodles, mix well, and cook for another 2 minutes or until the noodles are soft and the chicken completely cooked.

6. Transfer to your serving plates, sprinkle with Parmesan cheese and serve.

Nutrition: Calories 179, Fat 8,5, Fiber 2,2, Carbs 8,5, Protein 19,3.

18.   Chicken Spring Onion Cream

Preparation Time: 10 minutes

Cooking Time: 20 minutes

Servings: 4

Ingredients:

- 1 ½ lb of boneless chicken breasts (skinless and pounded to ⅜ inch thick)
- 1 teaspoon of a mix of sea salt and black pepper
- 1 cup of chicken broth (low sodium)
- 2 teaspoons of fresh lemon juice
- 1 tablespoon of garlic and spring onion seasoning (or use a mixture of chives, fresh garlic, lemon, salt, and pepper)
- 4 tablespoons of low-fat cream cheese
- 2 tablespoons of butter
- To garnish, use parsley, lemon wedges, and/or fresh basil

Directions:

1. Grease the non-stick pan with cooking spray and place it over medium-high heat.

2. Season the chicken breast with a pinch of salt and pepper and as soon as the pan has heated up, place the chicken on top and cook on each side for about 6 minutes.

3. Add the lemon juice, broth, and garlic dressing to the pan and mix well to combine.

4. Scrape the brown bits from the bottom of the pan with the spatula and simmer for another 12 minutes or until the sauce is reduced to a third of a cup.

5. Add the butter and cream cheese to the pan and mix until smooth.

6. Remove from the heat and garnish with fresh lemon wedges, basil, or other aromatic herbs of your choice, serve and enjoy.

Nutrition: Calories 285, Fat 13,5, Fiber 0,1, Carbs 1,3, Protein 37,1.

19. Chicken Tuscan Caprese

Preparation Time: 10 minutes

Cooking Time: 25 minutes

Servings: 4

Ingredients:

- 4 teaspoons roasted garlic oil (or oil of your choice and fresh garlic)

- 1 ½ lb of boneless chicken breasts (skinless and pounded to ⅜ inch thick)

- 2 teaspoons of Tuscan seasoning (or use a mixture of parsley, garlic, black pepper, onion, red pepper, and garlic powder)

- 1 cup of Tomatoes (chopped)

- 8 tablespoons (1/2 cup) of low-fat mozzarella cheese (shredded)

- To garnish, use fresh basil.

Directions:

1. Preheat the oven to 350 degrees.

2. In a skillet, add the oil to heat over medium-high heat on a stove.

3. Season the chicken breasts with the Tuscan dressing and, once the oil has heated up, place the chicken in the pan and cook for 6 minutes on each side.

4. Place the chicken in an oven dish with the cherry tomatoes and sprinkle with the mozzarella and a pinch of Tuscan seasoning.

5. Place in the oven and cook for 10 minutes or until the chicken is cooked through.

6. Remove from the oven, garnish with fresh basil, and serve hot.

Nutrition: Calories 262, Fat 7.3, Fiber 0,5, Carbs 1,8, Protein 43,5.

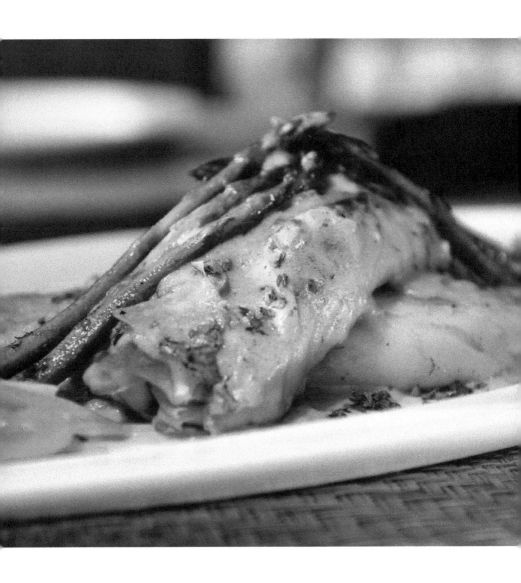

20. Creamy Chicken Asparagus

Preparation Time: 10 minutes

Cooking Time: 15 minutes

Servings: 4

Ingredients:

- 4 teaspoons of roasted garlic oil (or oil of your choice and fresh garlic)

- 1 3/4 lbs boneless chicken breast (skinless, and chopped into 1-inch chunks)

- ½ cup of chicken broth (low sodium)

- 1 tablespoon of garlic and spring onion seasoning (or use parsley, fresh garlic, and chives)

- 8 tablespoon of light cream cheese

- 4 cups of fresh asparagus (chopped into 2-inch pieces)

- Seasoning (salt, garlic, and pepper)

Directions:

1. Add the oil to the pan and heat it over medium-high heat.

2. Add the chicken breast and cook for about 10 minutes or until the chicken is lightly browned, turning occasionally.

3. Add the chicken broth to the pan and scrape all the brown bits from the bottom of the pan.

4. Add the garlic dressing, asparagus, and cream cheese.

5. Increase the heat to high and cook until the cream cheese melts completely stir frequently.

6. Bring the mixture to a boil and then simmer until the sauce thickens.

7. Divide equally into 4 portions, sprinkle with the dressing, and serve hot.

Nutrition: Calories 302, Fat 12,8, Fiber 2,8, Carbs 7,1, Protein 39.

21.   Curry Chicken And Cauliflower

Preparation Time: 10 minutes

Cooking Time: 15 minutes

Servings: 4

Ingredients:

- 1 tablespoon of roasted garlic oil (or another oil, with fresh garlic)
- 1 ½ pound of boneless chicken breast (skinless)
- 1 tablespoon of curry powder
- 4 cups of cauliflower florets
- 1 ½ cup of light coconut milk
- Ground pepper and natural sea salt - to taste

Directions:

1. Slice the chicken and set it aside.

2. Cut the cauliflower into ½ inch florets.

3. In a pan, add oil and garlic and heat over high heat to brown, then add the chicken and sprinkle with curry, mix well and cook for about 5 min.

4. Add the coconut milk and cauliflower, cover, and cook for about 10 minutes, until the chicken is completely cooked with the tender cauliflower.

5. Season with pepper and salt and serve.

Nutrition: Calories 231, Fat 5,4, Fiber 2,5, Carbs 6,3, Protein 38.

22.   Fall Chicken Noodle Stir Fry

Preparation Time: 10 minutes

Cooking Time: 5 minutes

Servings: 2

Ingredients:

*   4oz Trifecta chicken breast, diced into squares
*   ½ cup of butternut squash cubes, precooked
*   2 eggs, whole, scrambled
*   2oz of brown rice pad Thai Noodles
*   1 bspt of fish sauce
*   2 tsp sesame oil, untoasted
*   2 tbsp of Teriyaki Sauce
*   1 tbsp of sriracha
*   2 tsp of garlic
*   1 serving of fresh bean sprouts
*   Fresh cilantro for garnish
*   Red pepper flakes for garnish

Directions:

1. Cook the Pad Thai noodles as indicated by the package. Drain and kepp warm.

2. Heat up the pre-cooked butternut squash in the microwave. Cook for 3-5 minutes or until the squash softens.

3. In a non-stick skillet, heat up the oil over medium heat, add the garlic, Trifecta chicken, butternut squash and cut up the chicken in the skillet and heat until golden.

4. Add the eggs to the skillet and scramble.

5. As the noodles become 75%-80% cooked through, add to the skillet the noodles, the fish sauce, teriyaki sauce, and sriracha and stir often.

6. Add the bean sprouts and cook for an additional minute to two until bean sprouts are heated through.

7. Serve on a bowl and Top with red pepper flakes and cilantro.

23.   Ginger Chicken and Noodles

Preparation Time: 5 minutes

Cooking Time: 20 minutes

Servings: 4

Ingredients:

- 4 tsp of orange oil
- 1 tablespoon of Thai seasoning (or use a mixture of any of orange zest, garlic, lime, ginger, lemongrass, onion, salt, red pepper, and pepper)
- 1 lime (juice)
- 1 ½ ls of boneless, chicken breasts (skinless, and cut in half)
- 4 cups of zucchini noodles (cooked)

Directions:

1. Add the oil, dressing, and lime juice to a plastic bag and massage to blend well.

2. Add the chicken to the marinade and let the air out of the bag.

3. Seal the bag tightly and let it rest in the refrigerator for about 4 hours or overnight.

4. Preheat the grill, place the chicken on the grill, and cook both sides of the chicken over medium-high heat for about 15 minutes each, or until the chicken is well cooked.

5. Serve the chicken over the zucchini noodles.

Nutrition: Calories 252, Fat 9, Fiber 1,2, Carbs 3,8, Protein 37,4.

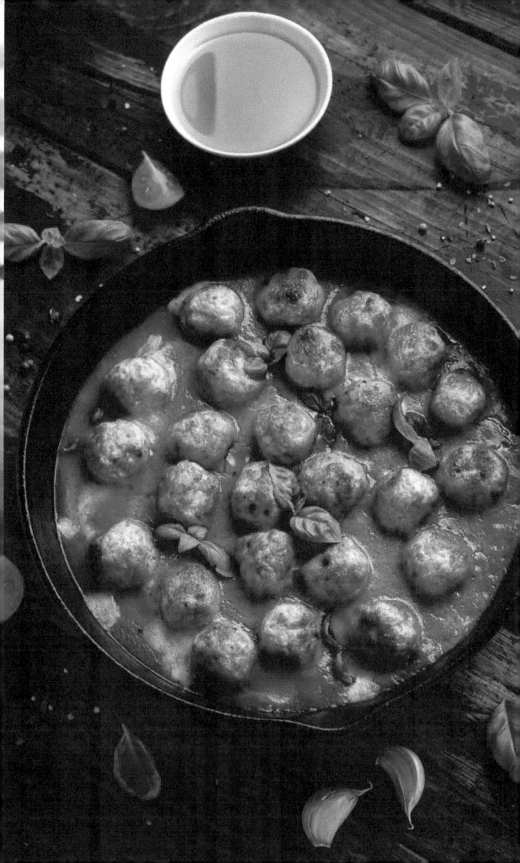

24. High Protein Chicken Meatballs

Preparation Time: 5 minutes

Cooking Time: 25 minutes

Servings: 2

Ingredients:

- 1 lb of chicken(lean, ground)

- ¾ cups of oats rolled

- 2 onions, grated

- 2 tsp of allspice, ground

- Salt and black pepper

Directions:

1. Heat a large skillet over medium heat and grease it using cooking spray.

2. In a large-sized bowl, add in the onions (grated), chicken (lean, ground), oats (rolled), allspice (earth), and a dash of salt and black pepper and stir well.

3. From the mixture make small meatballs and place them into the skillet.

4. Cook for roughly 5 minutes until golden brown on all sides, then remove meatballs from heat, serve immediately and enjoy!

Nutrition: Calories 519, Fat 15, Carbs 32, Protein 57.

25. Instant Pot Chipotle Chicken & Cauliflower Rice Bowls

Preparation Time: 10 minutes

Cooking Time: 20 minutes

Servings: 4

Ingredients:

- 1/3 cup of salsa

- quantity of 14.5 oz. of can fire-roasted diced tomatoes

- 1 canned chipotle pepper + 1 teaspoon sauce

- ½ teaspoon of dried oregano

- 1 teaspoon of cumin

- 1 ½ lb. of boneless, skinless chicken breast

- ¼ teaspoon of salt

- 1 cup of reduced-fat shredded Mexican cheese blend

- 4 cups of frozen riced cauliflower

- ½ medium-sized avocado, sliced

Directions:

1. Combine the first ingredients in a blender and blend until the mixture is smooth

---

2. Place the chicken in the Instant Pot and pour the sauce over it.

3. Cover with the lid, close the pressure valve and set it to 20 minutes at a high temperature.

4. Let the pressure release on its own before opening, then remove the chicken and add it back to the sauce.

5. Meanwhile, microwave the cauliflower following package directions.

6. Divide the cauliflower, cheese, avocado, and chicken equally among the four bowls, serve, and enjoy.

Nutrition: Calories 287, Fiber 12, Carbs 19, Protein 35.

26. Lemon Garlic Oregano Chicken with Asparagus

Preparation Time: 5 minutes

Cooking Time: 40 minutes

Servings: 4

Ingredients:

- 1 small lemon, juiced (this should be about 2 tablespoons of lemon juice)

- 1 ¾ lb. of bone-in, skinless chicken thighs

- 2 tablespoons of fresh oregano, minced

- 2 cloves of garlic, minced

- 2 lbs. of asparagus, trimmed

- ¼ teaspoon each or less of black pepper and salt

Directions:

1. Preheat the oven to about 350 ° F.

2. Place the chicken in a medium-sized bowl, add the garlic, oregano, lemon juice, pepper, and salt, and mix.

3. Roast the chicken in the oven or air fryer until it reaches a core temperature of 165 ° F in about 40 minutes.

4. Once the chicken legs are cooked, remove them, and set aside warm.

5. Steam the asparagus on a stovetop or in a microwave until cooked through.

6. Serve the asparagus with the roasted chicken legs and enjoy.

Nutrition: Calories 350, Fat 10, Carbs 10, Protein 32.

27.   Mixed Veggie Chicken Kebabs

Preparation Time: 5 minutes

Cooking Time: 20 minutes

Servings: 8-10
Ingredients:
- 1 cup of onion slices
- ¼ cup of Chicken broth (low sodium)
- 4 tablespoon of balsamic vincotto (or use a balsamic reduction - do not use vinegar)
- Pinch of sea salt and fresh peppercorns

Directions:
1. In a pan, add the broth and onions and cook over medium heat for about 20 minutes without browning.

2. When the onions have become soft, add the balsamic vinegar.

3. Turn off the stove and stir gently; let the onions soak in the balsamic and then serve.

Note: Can be stored in the refrigerator for up to 1 week.

Nutrition: Calories 6, Fat 0, Fiber 0,2, Carbs 1,4, Protein 0,1.

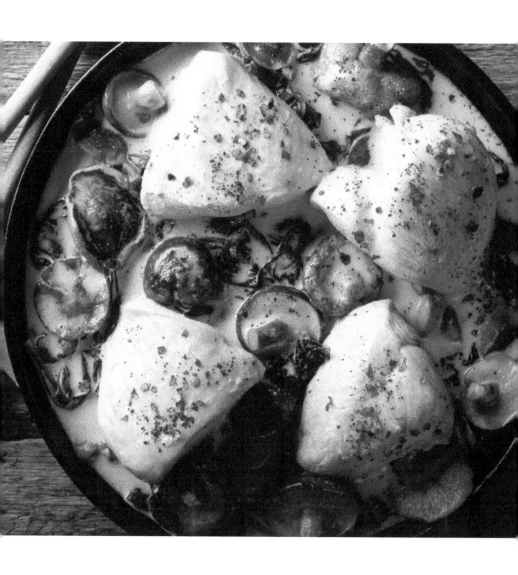

28. Mushrooms Chicken

Preparation Time: 10 minutes

Cooking Time: 15 minutes

Servings: 4

Ingredients:

- ½ cup of chicken broth (low sodium)
- 1 ½ lb of chicken tenderloins (cut into 1-inch chunks)
- 1 tablespoon of garlic gusto seasoning (or use a mixture of parsley, garlic, lemon, onion, and paprika)
- 4 cups of sliced mushrooms
- 1 ½ teaspoon of Alderwood smoked sea salt (or use any smoke seasoning such as liquid smoke)
- 2 tablespoons of butter

Directions:

1. Add the broth to a skillet and heat over medium-high heat until it starts to boil.

2. Add the chicken, sprinkle with the garlic dressing and cook for about 4 minutes, stirring occasionally.

3. Add the mushrooms and cook for another 8 minutes or until the chicken is completely cooked and most of the liquid has evaporated.

4. Add the butter and stir until completely melted, scraping any brown bits from the bottom of the pan.

5. Sprinkle the mixture with sea salt, serve, and enjoy.

Nutrition: Calories 201, Fat 4,4, Fiber 0,4, Carbs 1,2, Protein 37,2.

29. Mustard Chicken Broccoli

Preparation Time: 5 minutes

Cooking Time: 25 minutes

Servings: 5
Ingredients:
- 1 tablespoon of Dijon mustard
- 1 tablespoon of whole-grain mustard
- 1 cup of low-sodium chicken broth
- 4 tsp of roasted garlic oil (or use another oil and fresh garlic)
- 4 cups of broccoli florets (fresh)
- 1 tablespoon of garlic gusto seasoning
- 1 ½ lb of boneless chicken breasts (skinless)
- A pinch of seasoning (or use onion, salt, garlic, pepper, and parsley)

Directions:
1. Add the broth and mustard to a bowl and whisk well.

2. Heat the oil in a skillet over medium-high heat, add the broccoli and seasoning and cook for about 2 minutes, stirring to coat well.

3. Transfer the cooked broccoli to a bowl.

4. Add the chicken to the pan and cook each side for about 5 minutes, then turn the heat down to medium and pour the broth mixture into the pan.

---

5. Add the broccoli, cover the pan and simmer for about 7 minutes or until the chicken is well cooked.

6. Remove from heat, sprinkle with a dressing, and serve.

Nutrition: Calories 277, Fat 9,4, Fiber 2,7, Carbs 7,4, Protein 39,6.

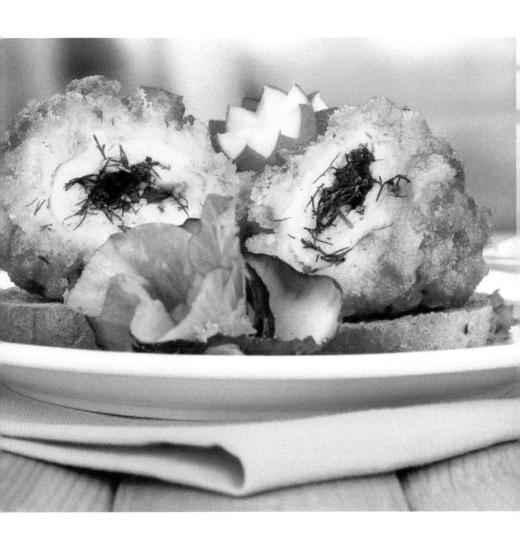

30. Roasted Chicken Dill Radishes

Preparation Time: 5 minutes

Cooking Time: 30 minutes

Servings: 4

Ingredients:
- 2 lbs of skinless chicken thighs
- A pinch of seasoning of choice (or a mixture of garlic, parsley, salt, black pepper, and onion)
- 1 tablespoon of Mediterranean seasoning (or a mixture of basil, garlic, rosemary, marjoram, and onion)

Directions:
1. Preheat the oven to 375 degrees.

2. Season the chicken legs and place the chicken in the pan without touching.

3. Sprinkle the Mediterranean dressing and bake for about 30 minutes.

4. Remove from the oven, serve, and enjoy!

Nutrition: Calories 269, Fat 10,5, Fiber 0, Carbs 0, Protein 41.

31.   Rosemary Trimmed-Pork Loin

Preparation Time: 5 minutes

Cooking Time: 25 minutes

Servings: 4

Ingredients:
- 1 ½ pound of thin-sliced boneless, skinless pork loin (trim out all excess fat)

- 1 tablespoon of rosemary seasoning (or garlic, rosemary, parsley, onion, black pepper, sage, thyme, salt)

- 4 teaspoons of Roasted garlic oil (or garlic, and oil of your choice)

Directions:
1. Preheat the oven to 375 degrees.

2. Add the oil and seasoning to a bowl and mix well.

3. Dry the pork loin and distribute the seasoning evenly on one side of the pork loin pieces.

4. Place the seasoned pork chops in a roasting pan, place in the oven, and cook for about 25 minutes, or until the temperature of the pork reaches 150 degrees.

5. Transfer the pork to a plate and let it cool for about 5 minutes and then serve.

Nutrition: Calories 283, Fat 10,5, Fiber 0, Carbs 0, Protein 44,5.

32. Scampi Chicken Noodles

Preparation Time: 5 minutes

Cooking Time: 10 minutes

Servings: 4

Ingredients:

- 1 ½ lb of boneless chicken breast (skinless and cut into thin slices)

- 1-2 tablespoons of Scampi seasoning (or onion, fresh garlic, lemon, pepper, parsley, and salt)

- 4 cups of green zucchini noodles

- 4 tsp of lemon oil (or another oil and lemon zest)

- A pinch of Seasoning (or salt, pepper, onion, garlic, and parsley)

Directions:

1. Into a bowl, add the chicken and sprinkle very well with the sauce for the scampi.

2. In a skillet, add the oil and heat over medium-high heat.

3. Add the chicken and cook for about 10 minutes or until the chicken is cooked through, stirring occasionally.

4. Transfer the chicken to a bowl and cover it to keep warm.

5. Add the zucchini to the pan, sauté for a minute and sprinkle with the dressing.

6. Add the chicken to the pan, mix well, and serve.

Nutrition: Calories 284, Fat 9,7, Fiber 1,2, Carbs 3,8, Protein 43,4.

33. Sesame Chicken

Preparation Time: 10 minutes

Cooking Time: 15 minutes

Servings: 4
Ingredients:
- 4 teaspoons of orange oil (or use any other oil and orange zest)
- 1 ½ lb of boneless chicken breast (skinless)
- 1 tablespoon of toasted sesame ginger seasoning (or use toasted sesame seeds, ground ginger, garlic, red pepper, salt, onion powder, pepper, and lemon)

Directions:
1. Place the chicken breast on a cutting board, flatten it to ⅜ inch thick with the meat tenderizer and sprinkle with the seasoning.

2. In a skillet, add the orange oil and heat over medium-high heat.

3. Add the chicken and cook each side for about 8 minutes or until the chicken is well cooked and then serve.

Nutrition: Calories 247, Fat 9,9, Fiber 0,3, Carbs 0,5, Protein 36,5.

34. Sheet Pan Chicken Fajita Lettuce Wraps

Preparation Time: 15 minutes

Cooking Time: 30 minutes

Servings: 2

Ingredients:

- 1 lb. chicken breast, thinly sliced into strips

- 2 teaspoon of olive oil

- 2 bell peppers, thinly sliced into strips

- 2 teaspoon of fajita seasoning

- 6 leaves from a romaine heart

- Juice of half a lime

- ¼ cup plain of non-fat Greek yogurt

Directions:

1. Preheat the oven to about 400°F.

2. Combine all ingredients (except lettuce) in a large plastic bag; close it and mix very well to coat vegetables and chicken with oil and seasoning evenly.

3. Distribute the contents of the bag evenly on a tin lined with aluminum foil. Cook for about 25-30 minutes, until the chicken is fully cooked.

4. Serve on lettuce leaves and garnish with Greek yogurt if desired.

Nutrition: Calories 387, Fat 6, Carbs 14, Protein 18.

35. Slow Cooker Jamaican Chicken Stew

Preparation Time: 5 minutes

Cooking Time: 20 minutes

Servings: 8-10

Ingredients:

- 3 lb chicken parts
- 2 tsp curry powder
- 1 ½ tsp dried thyme
- ¾ tsp ground allspice
- ½ tsp red pepper flakes
- ½ tsp black pepper
- ½ tsp salt
- 2 tsp olive oil
- 1 medium onion chopped
- 3 cloves garlic minced
- ½ c. red wine
- 1 ½ c. 15 ounces black beans, rinsed and drained
- 1 ½ c. 15 ounces diced tomatoes, undrained

Directions:

1. Season chicken with curry powder, thyme, allspice, red pepper flakes, black pepper and salt.

2. In a large skillet, heat oil; add onions and garlic and sauté until onions are softened, about 3 minutes.

3. Add chicken mixture to skillet and brown on both sides, then add wine and let cook for a few minutes.

4. Add tomatoes and black beans and mix well.

5. Transfer to crock pot and cook in high for 4-5 hours until tender and meat is falling off the bone. Alternatively, you can continue to cook the chicken on the stove top for about 25-30 minutes until chicken is done.

6. Serve and enjoy!

Nutrition: Calories 423, Fat 24, Fiber 4, Carbs 13, Protein 32.

36. Taco Sunrise Seasoned Chicken

Preparation Time: 5 minutes

Cooking Time: 10 minutes

Servings: 4

Ingredients:

- 1 ½ pound of boneless chicken breast (skinless)
- 1 tablespoon of phoenix sunrise seasoning (or use any low salt tex-mix seasoning)
- ½ cup of fresh tomatoes (chopped)
- 1 tsp of Seasoning
- Favorite taco condiments

Directions:

1. At the bottom of an Instant Pot, place the chicken slices in a single layer.

2. Sprinkle the chicken with seasonings and spread the tomatoes over the chicken.

3. Close the lid, seal the vent, and cook over high heat for 9 minutes and quick release.

4. Remove the chicken from the pot, chop with forks, pour the sauce over the chicken and serve.

Nutrition: Calories 198, Fat 4,3, Fiber 0,3, Carbs 0,9, Protein 36,3.

37. Tomato Braised Cauliflower with Chicken

Preparation Time: 10 minutes

Cooking Time: 30 minutes

Servings: 4

Ingredients:

- 4 garlic cloves, sliced

- 3 scallions, to be trimmed and cut into 1-inch pieces

- ¼ teaspoon of dried oregano

- ¼ teaspoon of crushed red pepper flakes

- 4 ½ cups of cauliflower

- 1 ½ cups of diced canned tomatoes

- 1 cup of fresh basil, gently torn

- ½ teaspoon each of pepper and salt, divided

- 1 ½ teaspoon of olive oil

- 1 ½ lb. of boneless, skinless chicken breasts

Directions:

1. In a saucepan, combine the garlic, shallot, oregano, chopped red pepper, cauliflower, tomato, and add ¼ cup of water.

2. Boil everything together and add ¼ teaspoon of pepper and salt for seasoning, then cover the pot with a lid.

3. Leave to simmer for 10 minutes and stir as often as possible until the cauliflower is tender, then season with the remaining ¼ teaspoon of pepper and salt.

4. Season the chicken breast with olive oil and roast it in the oven at 450 °F for 20 minutes and a core temperature of 165 °F.

5. Remove from the oven and allow the chicken to rest for about 10 minutes, then slice the chicken and serve on a bed of tomato-braised cauliflower.

Nutrition: Calories 400, Fat 20, Carbs 11, Protein 44.

38.   Tuscan Baked Chicken

Preparation Time: 5 minutes

Cooking Time: 30 minutes

Servings: 4

Ingredients:

- 1 ¾ pound of boneless chicken thighs
- Seasoning of choice (or red pepper, black pepper, lemon, garlic, oregano, thyme, salt, onion, parsley, and marjoram)

Directions:

1. Preheat the oven to 375 degrees.

2. In a baking dish, arrange the chicken legs apart so that they do not touch each other.

3. Sprinkle evenly with the sauce and bake for about 35 minutes.

4. Remove from the oven and transfer to a serving dish.

5. Leave to cool for about 5 minutes before serving.

Nutrition: Calories 269, Fat 10,5, Fiber 0, Carbs 0, Protein 41.

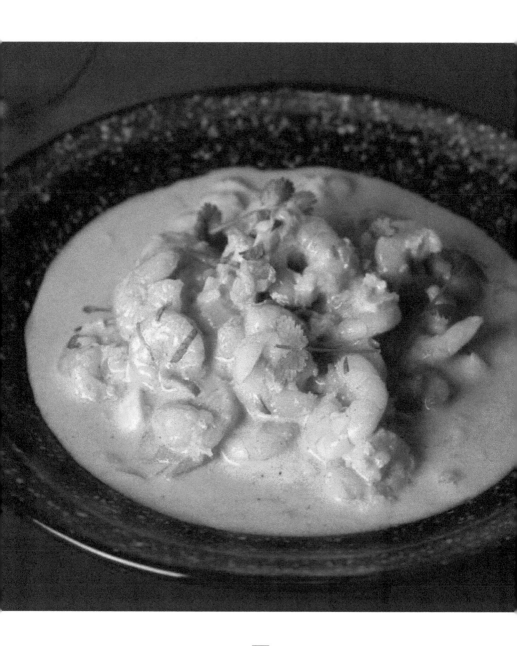

39. Shrimp Curry

Preparation Time: 15 minutes

Cooking Time: 20 minutes

Servings: 4
Ingredients:

- 2 tablespoons of peanut oil

- ¼ onion

- 2 cloves garlic

- 1 teaspoon ginger

- 1 teaspoon cumin

- 1 teaspoon turmeric

- 1 teaspoon paprika

- ¼ red chili powder

- 1 can tomatoes

- 1 can coconut milk

- 1 lb. peeled shrimp

- 1 tablespoon cilantro

Directions:
1. In a skillet, add onion and cook for 4-5 minutes.

2. Add ginger, cumin, garlic, chili, and paprika, and cook on low heat for a few minutes.

3. Pour the tomatoes and the coconut milk and simmer for 10-12 minutes.

4. Add in shrimp and cilantro, and cook them for 2-3 minutes stirring slowly.

5. Serve and enjoy!

Nutrition: Calories 178, Fat 17, Carbs 3, Protein 9.

40.   Shrimp Primavera

Preparation Time: 10 minutes

Cooking Time: 10 minutes

Servings: 4

Ingredients:

- 4 teaspoons of lemon or roasted garlic oil
- 2 pounds of raw shrimp (wild-caught, peeled, and deveined)
- 1 tablespoon of garlic and spring onion seasoning (or use sea salt, fresh garlic, scallions, parsley, and lemon)
- ½ cup of chicken broth (low sodium)
- 6 cups of vegetable noodles
- 1 scallion green tops (sliced for garnish)
- 8 tablespoons of fresh parmesan cheese (grated for garnish)

Directions:

1. Using vegetable peelers make the noodles, then set them aside in a bowl.

2. In a pan, heat the oil over medium-high heat, and then add shrimp and cook them on each side for about 4 minutes.

3. Sprinkle the seasoning over them and cook for an extra 3 min.

4. Deglaze the pan by adding the broth and cook for another 2 min, or until the shrimp is well cooked.

5. Remove the shrimp and put it into a bowl, then return the pan to the heat and cook until the liquid starts to bubble.

6. Add the vegetable noodles and saute for about 2 minutes, until crisp and tender.

7. Finally transfer the noodles into a platter, top with the cooked shrimp, sprinkle over with the parmesan cheese and scallions, and serve hot! Enjoy!

Nutrition: Calories 281, Fat 9, Fiber 0,2, Carbs 3,4, Protein 44.

CPSIA information can be obtained
at www.ICGtesting.com
Printed in the USA
BVHW051447220321
603178BV00010B/658